DEFEATING CROHN'S DISEASE WITH EXPERT GUIDANCE

Ultimate Solution Handbook For Patients, Guardians Or Family To Understand, Manage, Treat, Prevent, Reverse Symptoms And Live Well

DR. POTTER WHITLEY

DISCLAIMER:

This book's contents are meant to be used solely for informative purposes. The information should not be used as a replacement for expert medical advice, diagnosis, or care.

The information contained in this book is accurate and reliable, having been verified by the author to the best of his ability. Nevertheless, thc author disclaims all express and implied representations and warranties regarding the availability, correctness, appropriateness, completeness, and reliability of the material provided here. You bear full responsibility for any reliance you may have on such material.

For informational purposes, this book may make reference to or mention of certain people, things, websites, organizations, or other names. The author has no connection to, endorsement from, or recommendation for these organizations.

The author's approval or validation is not implied by the inclusion of these references.

Any direct, indirect, incidental, special, or consequential damages resulting from using or not being able to use the material in this book are not covered by the author's liability policy. For medical advice and counsel particular to their circumstances, readers are advised to check with experienced healthcare specialists.

The content, materials, and information in this book are subject to change at any time without prior notice, at the author's discretion. The text may contain errors or omissions for which the author is not responsible.

By reading this book, you understand and accept the conditions of this disclaimer.

THE REASON BEHIND THIS BOOK

For those battling the intricacies of Crohn's disease, "Defeating Crohn's Disease With Expert Guidance" is a source of empowerment and understanding. This book begins with a thorough introduction that provides a sophisticated synopsis of the condition and highlights the critical role that professional advice plays in its management. This book builds a strong foundation by exploring the complexities of Crohn's disease in the first few chapters, making sure readers understand the nuances of the disease's definition, types, causes, and diagnostic procedures.

This book's thorough examination of the role that nutrition and diet play in managing Crohn's disease is one of its best features. Acknowledging the crucial part these elements play in managing symptoms, this book offers certain dietary plans and precise nutritional recommendations. By exploring holistic techniques and embracing integrative medicine, complementary therapies, and the mind-body link, it goes beyond traditional medical procedures.

The addition of stress reduction techniques, yoga, and meditation emphasizes a holistic approach to wellbeing that goes beyond conventional medical paradigms.

This book guides readers through a variety of drug alternatives, surgical procedures, and cutting-edge therapies in the field of medical treatments. People are not only empowered to make knowledgeable decisions about their healthcare journey but they are also informed. A remarkable part of the value of exercise emphasizes how important it is to manage Crohn's disease by customizing workout regimens to meet each person's needs for maximum well-being.

A recurring subject is the need to have a strong support network, which instructs readers on how to create one that includes friends, family, and professional counseling. This book deftly negotiates the healthcare system, providing guidance on selecting the best medical team, communicating with providers, and comprehending insurance and budgetary issues.

For those with Crohn's disease, useful advice on overcoming obstacles, managing everyday tasks, and striking a balance between job and health serves as a road map. Real-life accounts from people who have overcome Crohn's disease provide a human touch and inspire resiliency and hope. Inspiring readers to imagine a time when Crohn's disease is better understood and treated more successfully, this book looks ahead at research, advancements, and campaigning.

"Defeating Crohn's Disease With Expert Guidance" goes above what is often expected of a medical manual by providing a comprehensive method for managing and curing Crohn's disease in addition to knowledge. For individuals impacted by Crohn's disease, this book proves to be a vital ally on their path to improved health and well-being because of its lively style and thoughtful treatment of important subjects.

TABLE OF CONTENT

CHAPTER ONE

OVERVIEW
An Outline Of Crohn's Disease

Every area of the gastrointestinal system, including the mouth and the anus, can be impacted by Crohn's disease, a chronic inflammatory bowel illness. It is typified by deep-seated inflammation in the intestinal tissue, which can cause a variety of symptoms including diarrhea, exhaustion, weight loss, and abdominal discomfort.

This illness is renowned for its erratic behavior, exhibiting periods of remission interspersed with flare-ups. Although the precise etiology of Crohn's disease is still unknown, a mix of immune system, environmental, and genetic variables are thought to be involved.

The capacity of Crohn's disease to affect several layers of the gastrointestinal tract and cause problems such as strictures, fistulas, and abscesses is one of its distinguishing characteristics. Beyond the digestive tract, other areas of the body such as the joints, skin, and eyes can also be affected by the inflammation linked to Crohn's disease. Because of its wide range of symptoms, which frequently coincide with those of other gastrointestinal disorders, diagnosing Crohn's disease can be difficult. It can start at any age, but it usually does so in the early stages of adulthood.

A multidisciplinary strategy is necessary to manage Crohn's disease, and it entails medication, lifestyle changes, and, occasionally, surgery. Reducing inflammation, easing symptoms, and enhancing the patient's quality of life are the objectives of treatment. However, because the disease is specific and patients respond differently to different therapies, developing an efficient and individualized treatment plan can be a challenging procedure.

Research endeavors are concentrated on discovering new therapy targets and enhancing diagnostic instruments as our comprehension of Crohn's disease keeps developing. Beyond just physical symptoms, the condition influences patients' emotional health and day-to-day functioning. Consequently, providing complete care for people with Crohn's disease entails attending to not just the physical but also the psychological and dietary aspects of their lives.

The Value of Professional Advice in Treatment:

Healthcare providers with expertise in gastroenterology and inflammatory bowel illnesses are essential in navigating the intricacies of Crohn's disease. It is impossible to exaggerate the value of professional advice when treating Crohn's disease because these experts have the skills and understanding required to customize treatment regimens to meet the specific requirements of each patient.

Accurate diagnosis is the first step toward expert assistance, and it may need a mix of laboratory testing, imaging studies, and clinical assessment. Because they are skilled at differentiating Crohn's disease from other gastrointestinal disorders, gastroenterologists with experience managing the disease can make sure that patients receive prompt and focused therapies. This is essential to avoiding treatment initiation delays, which can have a serious negative effect on the patient's general health and the course of the disease.

Following diagnosis, the degree of inflammation, the patient's general health, and the intensity of the symptoms are all taken into account by an expert-guided treatment plan. To address the various components of Crohn's disease, gastroenterologists work in conjunction with a multidisciplinary team that includes surgeons, psychiatrists, and nutritionists. By combining medical and lifestyle therapies, this cooperative strategy seeks to maximize treatment efficacy and raise patient quality of life.

Since gastroenterologists are knowledgeable about the most recent developments in the treatment of inflammatory bowel disease, their advice is especially helpful when it comes to medication management. They are adept at navigating the variety of available drugs, including biologics, immunosuppressants, and corticosteroids, and they can customize treatment plans to optimize effectiveness while lowering the risk of side effects.

In addition, professional advice goes beyond the therapeutic context to include patient assistance and education. When it comes to educating patients about their disease, encouraging self-management, and offering support for managing the emotional difficulties that frequently accompany chronic conditions like Crohn's disease, gastroenterologists are essential.

With Crohn's disease, where every patient's story is different, professional advice provides a ray of hope. It fosters a cooperative and patient-centered approach to managing this chronic condition by giving people the confidence that their care is in the hands of experts who comprehend the nuances of the illness. As research on Crohn's disease advances, professional advice plays an increasingly important role in the quest for better results and a higher standard of living for those afflicted with this complicated condition.

CHAPTER TWO

COMPREHENDING CROHN'S DISEASE
Types and Definitions of Crohn's Disease:

An inflammatory bowel disease (IBD) that is persistent and can affect any region of the gastrointestinal tract, including the mouth and the anus, is called Crohn's disease. It is typified by intestinal tract lining destruction and inflammation, which can result in a variety of symptoms and problems. Although the precise origin of Crohn's disease is still unknown, a mix of immune system, environmental, and genetic variables are thought to be involved.

The site and pattern of inflammation in the digestive tract differentiate the various forms of Crohn's disease. The most prevalent kinds are jejunoileitis, which affects the upper half of the small intestine, gastroduodenal Crohn's disease, which affects the stomach and the beginning of the small intestine, ileocolitis, which affects both the large and end of the small intestine, and ileitis, which only affects the ileum. Crohn's disease is a complex and heterogeneous ailment because each person's kind and severity can differ.

Comprehending the various varieties is essential for customizing therapeutic strategies, as every subtype may exhibit unique obstacles and indications. For instance, gastroduodenal Crohn's disease may result in nausea, vomiting, and a fullness sensation, whereas ileocolitis frequently causes diarrhea, stomach pain, and weight loss. The fact that symptoms and affected areas vary so much highlights how crucial individualized therapy is for the management of Crohn's disease.

Reasons and Danger Factors:

Although the precise etiology of Crohn's disease is still unknown, it is generally acknowledged that a mix of immunological, environmental, and genetic variables play a role in the illness' development. The hereditary component of IBD is highlighted by the increased chance of getting the disorder in people with a family history of the illness, particularly Crohn's disease. There are some gene mutations associated with immune system function that may be involved in the disease.

A role may also be played by environmental variables like food, smoking, and prior infections. For example, smoking is a risk factor for Crohn's disease and can exacerbate the condition. Furthermore, the collection of bacteria in the digestive tract known as the gut microbiome is believed to have an impact on the onset and course of Crohn's disease.

People who are predisposed to Crohn's disease are thought to experience inflammation as a result of their immune system's reaction to normal gut microorganisms. The gastrointestinal system is harmed and persistent inflammation is the outcome of this aberrant immune response. The interaction and diversity of genetic and environmental variables make it difficult to identify a single cause, even though these components offer insightful information about the possible reasons.

Signs and Prognosis:

There are numerous ways that Crohn's disease presents itself, and they can impact various areas of the digestive system. Abdominal pain, diarrhea, exhaustion, weight loss, and in certain situations, rectal bleeding are typical symptoms. Nonetheless, there might be significant individual variation in the combination and intensity of symptoms.

An extensive approach involving a physical examination, a detailed medical history, and several diagnostic tests is required to diagnose Crohn's disease. Blood tests can be used to measure dietary deficits and inflammation. Imaging tests, which include colonoscopies, endoscopies, and imaging scans, enable medical practitioners to see within the digestive tract, spot inflammation, and take tissue samples for additional examination.

Eliminating illnesses like ulcerative colitis and irritable bowel syndrome (IBS) that present with similar symptoms is frequently necessary for a final diagnosis. Because Crohn's disease is so complex, a multidisciplinary approach comprising radiologists, pathologists, and gastroenterologists is essential for precise diagnosis and individualized therapy planning. For people with Crohn's disease to improve their quality of life and put into practice appropriate management techniques, an early and precise diagnosis is essential.

CHAPTER THREE

DIET AND NUTRITION'S ROLE
Dietary Influence on Crohn's Disease

The digestive system becomes inflamed with Crohn's disease, a chronic inflammatory bowel illness. Although there is no treatment for Crohn's disease, nutrition is extremely important for symptom management and enhancing general health in those who have it. Diet has a complex effect on Crohn's disease, affecting both the severity of flare-ups and when symptoms first appear.

A few food items may either cause or worsen Crohn's disease symptoms. For instance, consuming large amounts of lipids, such as trans and saturated fats, may aggravate intestinal inflammation. Similarly, some people may experience worsening symptoms while eating processed foods or foods heavy in refined sugars.

Furthermore, some people with Crohn's disease may have dietary sensitivity issues, such as dairy or gluten, which can worsen their discomfort and inflammation.

On the other hand, a diet low in inflammation can have a beneficial effect on managing Crohn's disease. Generally, this diet includes foods high in fiber, antioxidants, and omega-3 fatty acids, which can improve digestive health and reduce inflammation.

Whole grains, fruits, vegetables, and fish high in omega-3 fatty acids are frequently suggested as components of an anti-inflammatory diet. People with Crohn's disease must collaborate closely with dietitians and medical professionals to pinpoint particular food triggers and modify their eating patterns accordingly.

Furthermore, people with Crohn's disease must be properly hydrated because dehydration can worsen symptoms and lead to a drop in general health. To avoid difficulties, water intake should be closely watched, and electrolyte imbalances should be treated very well.

In conclusion, diet has a significant influence on Crohn's disease, with some foods having the ability to exacerbate symptoms while others help to control inflammation. People with Crohn's disease must take a tailored approach to eating under the direction of medical professionals to successfully manage the intricacies of diet.

Dietary Guidelines for Symptom Management

The management of Crohn's disease symptoms is significantly influenced by nutritional guidelines, which are designed to provide people with doable tactics to reduce pain, promote healing, and avoid malnourishment. These recommendations' major objectives are to minimize gastrointestinal discomfort, maintain an appropriate food intake, and enhance general well-being.

A crucial component of Crohn's disease nutritional management is keeping an eye on and modifying dietary fiber consumption. While a high-fiber diet may be beneficial for certain people, a low-fiber diet may be more beneficial for others in terms of symptom reduction and decreased digestive tract irritation. Based on each patient's unique requirements and tolerances, healthcare providers frequently collaborate with patients to identify the ideal dietary fiber intake.

Keeping an eye on your intake of macronutrients is just as important as fiber. Because protein is necessary for tissue upkeep and repair, people with Crohn's disease may require more protein when their inflammation is active. Maintaining overall nutritional health and supplying sustained energy require a balanced intake of fats and carbohydrates.

Another aspect of the dietary requirements for the management of Crohn's disease is supplementation. People may need more vitamins and minerals to prevent deficits because of possible malabsorption problems. B vitamins, calcium, iron, and vitamin D are common supplements. These supplements are frequently customized for each person's needs and may need to be changed in response to blood tests and symptom observation.

Furthermore, how often and when you eat can affect how you manage your symptoms. Larger, less frequent meals might not be as well tolerated as smaller, more frequent ones. Furthermore, maintaining a food journal can assist people in pinpointing particular triggers and trends associated with their symptoms, allowing for a more individualized and successful approach to nutritional management.

To summarize, nutritional guidelines for the management of Crohn's disease symptoms adopt a holistic approach, taking into account variables including fiber consumption, timing of meals, supplementation, and the balance of macronutrients. For people with Crohn's disease, these recommendations are crucial resources for improving their nutritional status and general quality of life.

Nutritional Approaches For Prolonged Well-Being

For those with Crohn's disease, long-term health depends on dietary approaches that are sustainable, manage symptoms, enhance general health, and avert complications. These tactics use a comprehensive approach to diet, taking into account both the maintenance of a healthy lifestyle and the immediate alleviation of symptoms.

The idea of "gentle" or readily digestible meals is central to long-term dietary treatments for Crohn's disease. These foods can be better tolerated during times of inflammation and are less likely to irritate the digestive tract. Lean proteins, cooked veggies, and thoroughly cooked grains are frequently suggested components of a moderate diet. The particulars of this diet, however, may differ from person to person, underscoring the significance of tailored advice from medical specialists.

For those with Crohn's disease, adding probiotics to the diet is another effective long-term treatment option. Probiotics, which are present in fermented foods and supplements, may help keep the proper balance of gut flora in the body, which may lower inflammation and improve digestive health. However, as every person reacts differently, selecting probiotics should be done in cooperation with medical professionals.

Long-term nutritional needs management for people with Crohn's disease also includes managing any side effects, such as vitamin shortages and bone health. Physicians can modify dietary advice and supplementation as necessary with routine monitoring through blood tests and other evaluations.

For those with Crohn's disease, eating in a mindful and stress-relieving manner is also essential to long-term health. Stress management practices, like yoga or meditation, can be added to dietary measures for better overall well-being. Stress has been associated with the worsening of symptoms in inflammatory bowel illnesses.

In summary, dietary solutions for long-term health in individuals with Crohn's disease need a comprehensive approach, taking into account elements like probiotics, easily digested meals, nutritional supplementation, and stress reduction.

Individuals with Crohn's disease can navigate their dietary path to promote prolonged well-being and manage the challenges of living with this chronic condition with regular advice from healthcare specialists.

CHAPTER FOUR

MEDICAL INTERVENTIONS
Drugs used to treat Crohn's disease

The digestive system is the main organ affected by Crohn's disease, a chronic inflammatory illness that manifests as lethargy, diarrhea, weight loss, and abdominal pain. A combination of dietary adjustments, medication, and lifestyle alterations is frequently used to control Crohn's disease. Using drugs to reduce inflammation and soothe symptoms is one of the mainstays of treating Crohn's disease.

Anti-inflammatory drugs, such as aminosalicylates, are the main class of medications used to treat Crohn's disease because they reduce inflammation in the digestive tract. During flare-ups, corticosteroids may also be administered to treat symptoms temporarily. However, continuous use is usually not advised due to the possibility of long-term negative effects.

Another class of drugs called immunomodulators works by inhibiting the immune system to lower inflammation. Methotrexate and thiopurines are two examples of immunomodulators that are frequently used to treat Crohn's disease.

Biologics, proteins created through genetic engineering to target particular immune system pathways, have completely changed how moderate-to-severe Crohn's disease is managed. This class of drugs includes adalimumab and infliximab.

The usefulness of pharmaceuticals varies from person to person, even though they are essential for managing Crohn's disease. Healthcare professionals frequently customize treatment regimens for each patient, taking into account the patient's general health as well as the disease's severity and particular symptoms.

Surgical Techniques and Operations:

Surgery may be required for certain Crohn's disease patients because the medicine may not be enough to relieve their symptoms. Whenever complications like abscesses, fistulas, or strictures (narrowing of the gut) occur, surgery is usually recommended.

Removing the impacted section of the intestine, reducing symptoms, and enhancing the patient's quality of life are the objectives of surgery for Crohn's disease.

Bowel resection is a frequently performed surgical surgery for Crohn's disease in which the diseased or damaged portion of the intestine is removed and the healthy ends are rejoined. People may need either a temporary or permanent ostomy, such as an ileostomy or colostomy, where a hole is made to redirect the flow of waste, in cases of severe inflammation and problems.

Surgery can help manage difficulties, but it's crucial to understand that it cannot treat Crohn's disease. There is still a chance for the illness to return in other digestive tract regions. Furthermore, people who have serious side effects or don't react well to medicine are usually the ones who need surgery.

New Research and Therapies:

The field of treating Crohn's disease is always changing, with research being done on new treatments and methods. Emerging therapies are intended to offer more specialized and efficient means of managing the illness, especially for those patients who might not react well to existing medications.

The creation of novel biologics that specifically target inflammatory process pathways is one area of ongoing research. Those with moderate to severe Crohn's disease may have new alternatives thanks to these innovative drugs. Furthermore, studies are being conducted to investigate the function of gut bacteria and the possibility of using microbiome-based treatments to reduce inflammation and reestablish a more balanced state in the digestive system.

Research on Crohn's disease is also beginning to emphasize personalized medicine. Through an understanding of the genetic and molecular features of a patient's sickness, medical professionals can customize therapy regimens to target particular underlying causes of the illness. This strategy has the potential to maximize therapeutic results while reducing adverse effects.

To sum up, the treatment landscape for Crohn's disease is always changing and involves many approaches such as medication, surgery, and continuous research into new therapies. The objective is still to give patients more individualized and efficient treatment options so they can manage and eventually overcome the difficulties brought on by Crohn's disease, even as our understanding of the condition grows.

CHAPTER FIVE

HOLISTIC METHODS FOR HANDLING CROHN'S DISEASE
Complementary Therapies And Integrative Medicine:

Integrative medicine and complementary therapies provide a comprehensive approach to managing Crohn's disease that goes beyond traditional medical interventions. Integrative medicine acknowledges the significance of treating a person's physical, emotional, and spiritual needs by fusing evidence-based traditional medicine with complementary therapies. Acupuncture, herbal supplements, and nutritional therapy are examples of complementary therapies that are effective in controlling Crohn's disease symptoms and enhancing general well-being.

The emphasis on customized treatment programs is one of the main tenets of integrative medicine. Together, patients and healthcare providers develop a comprehensive plan that is specific to their requirements and situation. This method tackles the underlying causes that may contribute to the onset and progression of Crohn's disease in addition to the illness's symptoms. Complementary therapies that target immune system regulation, inflammation reduction, and gut health optimization are frequently helpful in relieving patients.

For example, by encouraging improved energy flow throughout the body, the ancient Chinese medicine procedure of acupuncture has demonstrated potential in reducing Crohn's disease symptoms. Herbal remedies with anti-inflammatory qualities, such as aloe vera and turmeric, can support pharmacological treatments. Additionally, nutritional therapies work to enhance nutrient absorption and maintain gut health through targeted dietary modifications and supplements.

By incorporating these supplemental methods into traditional Crohn's disease care, patients are given more resources for managing their symptoms and are allowed to take an active role in their recovery. It gives them a sense of empowerment and encourages a deeper comprehension of the interrelated elements affecting their health.

The Mind-Body Link in Healing:

Understanding the complex relationship between the body and mind is crucial to managing Crohn's disease holistically. The trajectory of chronic illnesses, such as Crohn's disease and other inflammatory bowel diseases, is significantly influenced by the mind-body connection. Because the intensity and frequency of symptoms can be greatly influenced by stress, anxiety, and emotional variables, investigating mind-body therapies is essential to the whole management of illness.

A growing number of mindfulness-based interventions, including guided imagery and meditation, are being used to treat the psychosocial effects of Crohn's disease. By fostering awareness and acceptance, these techniques assist people in lessening the emotional toll that comes with having a chronic condition. Additionally, they aid in stress reduction, which is crucial for reducing flare-ups and preserving general well-being.

Cognitive-behavioral therapy (CBT), one type of psychotherapy, provides useful coping mechanisms for managing the emotional difficulties associated with having Crohn's disease. Patients gain the ability to recognize and alter harmful thought patterns, better handle stress, and strengthen their ability to bounce back from long-term sickness. The treatment plan's integration of psychotherapy approaches recognizes the multifaceted character of Crohn's disease and stresses the significance of treating mental health issues in addition to physical ones.

Individuals suffering from Crohn's disease might get a more harmonic and balanced attitude to their general health by accepting the mind-body link. Including these routines in daily life promotes emotional health, resilience, and a feeling of control over the obstacles the illness presents.

Meditation, Yoga, and Stress Reduction:

The integration of yoga, meditation, and stress-reduction practices is becoming increasingly popular in the holistic care of Crohn's disease as a means of fostering both mental and physical well-being. In addition to providing symptomatic relief, these strategies help those with Crohn's disease live more fully by proactively reducing flare-ups and improving their overall quality of life.

Yoga is a holistic exercise that addresses all elements of health because it combines physical postures, breath control, and meditation. Research indicates that consistent yoga practice helps lessen inflammation, enhance gastrointestinal health, and ease Crohn's disease symptoms. Yoga's focus on breath awareness and mindful movement encourages relaxation and helps with stress reduction, which is crucial for managing chronic diseases.

Another essential element is meditation, which offers a methodical way to calm the mind and develop inner serenity. Those who practice mindful meditation in particular are encouraged to watch their thoughts and feelings objectively, which promotes acceptance and emotional fortitude. Meditating helps people with Crohn's disease manage the psychological effects of their illness and reduce stressors that could worsen their symptoms.

The underlying concept of stress management acknowledges the substantial impact that stress has on the development of Crohn's disease. People can control their stress reactions by using methods like progressive muscle relaxation, biofeedback, and deep breathing techniques. Patients can foster an atmosphere that is more supportive of their general well-being and possibly lessen the frequency and severity of disease flare-ups by incorporating stress management into their everyday lives.

In conclusion, a proactive and powerful way for people to deal with the challenges of living with a chronic illness is provided by the integration of yoga, meditation, and stress management into the holistic approach to Crohn's disease management.

These methods promote mental and emotional fortitude in addition to treating the physical symptoms, creating a holistic approach to better health and vitality.

CHAPTER SIX

THE VALUE OF PHYSICAL ACTIVITY
The Relationship Between Exercise and Crohn's

A chronic inflammatory bowel disease that can seriously lower a person's quality of life is Crohn's disease. The significance of medication treatments in symptom management is critical, but it is as important to include regular physical exercise in the overall care strategy. Numerous facets of Crohn's disease have been demonstrated to benefit from exercise, including inflammation reduction, symptom relief, and general well-being enhancement.

Regular physical activity can help regulate the immune system, which is crucial for controlling the long-term inflammation linked to Crohn's disease. Pro- and anti-inflammatory cytokine balance has been shown to improve with exercise, as has the level of inflammatory markers. Thus, lessening the intensity of symptoms and frequency of flare-ups may be possible.

Additionally, exercise has been linked to increased gastrointestinal motility, which is important because people with Crohn's disease may have problems with their bowel movements.

Physical activity can help to maintain a more stable and predictable gastrointestinal function by encouraging regular bowel movements and improving the efficiency of the digestive process, which may lessen the influence of Crohn's symptoms on day-to-day living.

Exercise is essential for treating the psychological and emotional components of Crohn's disease in addition to its physiological advantages. People with the illness may face emotional difficulties and develop anxiety and sadness.

It has been demonstrated that regular physical activity improves mental health by lowering levels of stress, anxiety, and sadness. Given the complex interactions between physical and mental health in chronic illnesses like Crohn's disease, a holistic approach to well-being is particularly crucial.

Despite these advantages, it's crucial that people with Crohn's disease approach exercise with caution and collaborate closely with medical professionals to create a customized and secure exercise program. It's critical to recognize the restrictions and modify workout regimens to meet specific needs to avoid a possible worsening of symptoms. This customized strategy could entail altering the style, length, and intensity of exercise by the person's general fitness level, symptoms, and present state of health.

Customizing Workout Programs to Meet Personal Needs

For those with Crohn's disease, designing a successful fitness program necessitates a customized and meticulous approach. There isn't a single fitness regimen that works for everyone because this inflammatory bowel disease is different from other types. Rather, medical professionals—such as physical therapists and gastroenterologists—should work together to create customized strategies that take into account the unique requirements, constraints, and objectives of every individual.

Knowing how symptoms and disease activity vary from person to person with Crohn's disease is essential to designing fitness programs for them. A person's capacity for physical activity might be greatly impacted by flare-ups and remissions. Low-impact workouts like walking or mild yoga may be more appropriate during the disease's active phases, while a wider variety of exercises may be possible during remission.

It's also critical to take into account the possible influence of specific workout regimens on gastrointestinal issues. Some people may find that high-impact, high-intensity activities make their symptoms worse, while others may find them tolerable. It is essential to closely evaluate each person's response to various workouts and modify the regimen as necessary to avoid pain or consequences.

Moreover, fitness regimens must include flexibility and adaptability. Energy levels might vary, and fatigue is a common symptom of Crohn's disease. Consequently, it's critical to permit adjustments to exercise intensity and duration based on individual energy levels each day. Its flexibility guarantees that people can continue a regular workout regimen without going beyond their limitations when they're tired.

In conclusion, a key component of integrating physical activity into the care of Crohn's disease is customizing exercise regimens for each individual. This tailored strategy reduces the possibility of symptom exacerbation while also optimizing the possible benefits of exercise. People with Crohn's disease can use exercise to enhance their physical and emotional health by collaborating with medical providers and remaining aware of their bodies' specific demands.

CHAPTER SEVEN

BUILDING A SUPPORT SYSTEM
Family and Friends in the Journey

In the difficult fight against Crohn's disease, friends and family play a crucial role. Having a solid support system is essential because this chronic ailment can have an overwhelming mental and physical toll. Families frequently have to navigate uncharted ground, so having loved ones there no matter what can provide them with a sense of security and comfort.

Friends and family can help with everyday duties in a practical way, which can alleviate the symptoms of Crohn's disease for individuals who need them. Family support may make a big difference in easing the burden that people with this illness bear, whether it takes the form of listening, helping out around the house, or taking the person to medical appointments.

Furthermore, the compassion and empathy that friends and family can bring to the table can help cultivate a positive outlook, which is crucial for managing the emotional difficulties that come with having a chronic illness.

Furthermore, encouraging candid communication within the family can improve knowledge and comprehension of Crohn's disease. A more supportive atmosphere can be fostered by educating family members about the nature of the illness, its symptoms, and possible causes.

With this information, family members can make significant contributions to the patient's well-being and present a unified front against the complications of Crohn's disease.

Essentially, one should not tread the path of Crohn's disease alone. For those with Crohn's disease, having the steadfast support of family and friends not only improves their quality of life but also fortifies the relationships that help them get through the highs and lows of their health journey.

Taking Part in Support Groups

Crohn's disease is a complex terrain, and navigating it frequently takes more than simply the support of close friends and family. Getting involved in support groups designed specifically for people with this disease can be a game-changer when it comes to creating a thorough support network. These communities offer priceless forums for interacting with people who have gone through similar things, creating an unmatched sense of understanding and camaraderie.

People with Crohn's disease can share their experiences, trade coping mechanisms, and receive emotional support in support groups. Members form a connection via their common struggles and victories that go beyond virtual or in-person meeting spaces, offering a network of support that goes beyond the boundaries of organized get-togethers.

These communities also frequently act as archives for useful materials and information. Members exchange information about coping strategies, dietary guidelines, and the newest medical treatments, building a collective body of knowledge that might enable people to make wise health decisions. Not only does the reciprocal sharing of information among these groups help individuals who are directly impacted by Crohn's disease, but it also advances public knowledge and comprehension of the illness.

People who have Crohn's disease can benefit greatly from joining support groups. In addition to finding comfort in the experiences of others, these groups provide access to a wealth of collective wisdom that can help members overcome the problems presented by their chronic condition.

Expert Guidance and Support for Mental Health

Managing a chronic illness, such as Crohn's disease, can have an impact on one's mental and emotional health in addition to its physical symptoms. Getting help for mental health issues and professional counseling is essential for managing the psychological effects of having this illness.

Counseling offers a private, secure setting where people can communicate their worries, disappointments, and fears associated with Crohn's disease. A qualified mental health practitioner can assist patients in negotiating the emotional complications that come with having a chronic illness and help them create coping strategies to deal with the difficulties more skillfully.

Additionally, counseling can help people reframe how they see their situation, cultivate a more optimistic mindset, and give them the confidence to take back control of their lives. Because Crohn's disease is unpredictable, it can cause feelings of powerlessness. Developing adaptive techniques and resilience can be greatly aided by professional support.

Apart from individual counseling, group therapy sessions designed especially for people with chronic illnesses such as Crohn's disease can foster a sense of solidarity and mutual comprehension. In a supportive setting, these sessions enable participants to obtain important insights into managing the emotional effect of their health journey and to learn from each other's experiences.

To put it simply, incorporating mental health support and professional counseling into the overall care plan for people with Crohn's disease is a holistic approach that acknowledges and addresses the interdependence of mental and physical health. Making mental health a priority helps people develop a robust mindset, which in turn helps them be more resilient when dealing with the difficulties posed by Crohn's disease.

CHAPTER EIGHT

GETTING AROUND THE HEALTHCARE SYSTEM
Selecting the Appropriate Medical Team

Choosing the correct medical team is essential to effectively managing Crohn's disease. Due to the chronic condition's intricacy, a multidisciplinary approach including several medical providers is necessary. A comprehensive healthcare team for Crohn's disease must include gastroenterologists, trained nurses, nutritionists, and mental health professionals.

It's critical to select doctors who have experience managing inflammatory bowel illnesses (IBD), such as Crohn's disease. To find medical professionals with a track record of success, ask other members of the IBD community or your primary care physician for referrals.

Beyond knowledge, effective teamwork and communication are critical skills. Every facet of the illness, from psychological health to medical management, is attended to by a well-coordinated healthcare team.

Testimonials from patients and internet evaluations can offer important insights into how well healthcare practitioners get along with people. The healthcare team's accessibility should also be taken into account since timely coordination and communication are essential for handling unforeseen flare-ups and treatment modifications.

Patients need to assess the resources and support services that the medical team provides. Comprehensive care encompasses more than just medical care; it also includes support networks, educational materials, and help making lifestyle modifications. A comprehensive healthcare team helps the patient maintain a high quality of life in addition to treating the physical symptoms of Crohn's disease.

Efficient Interaction with Healthcare Professionals

Managing Crohn's disease requires open and efficient communication with medical professionals. Patients and their healthcare team should be at ease when discussing symptoms, treatment concerns, and lifestyle modifications. Frequent check-ins, whether in person or virtually, offer a chance to discuss any obstacles encountered and provide information on how the condition is progressing. Developing a close bond with medical professionals encourages a cooperative partnership in which patients take an active role in choosing their treatment.

Patients should make a list of their questions and concerns to prepare for their appointments. This proactive strategy guarantees that, in the brief amount of time allotted, pertinent issues are covered. Transparent communication goes beyond in-person exchanges and includes correspondence via email for non-urgent inquiries. Email communication options and patient portals are widely available to healthcare professionals, allowing for ongoing communication in between appointments.

Patients with Crohn's disease should describe how the illness affects their day-to-day activities, as symptoms might vary greatly. Talking about emotional and mental health issues is part of this since long-term conditions frequently have a significant impact on a patient's general well-being. Patients who communicate their physical and emotional problems to healthcare practitioners help them better customize treatment strategies, which improves Crohn's disease management overall.

Knowing About Insurance and Money Matters

One of the most important things in beating Crohn's disease is figuring out the financial side of things. Reducing the cost of continuing medical care requires an understanding of insurance coverage, copayments, and out-of-pocket costs. Patients should carefully go over their insurance plans to make sure they are covered for any necessary treatments, prescription drugs, and routine check-ups associated with Crohn's disease.

It is a good idea to find out from medical professionals how much of a given treatment is covered by insurance before beginning any kind of medical procedure. It may be necessary to obtain prior authorization for some treatments, particularly novel therapies, which calls for proactive discussion with insurance companies.

Additionally, patients should be informed about the nonprofit and pharmaceutical companies' financial assistance programs, which can help with the expense of prescription drugs.

When creating a budget for healthcare-related expenses, one must take into account not only the direct costs of care but also any possible indirect costs, such as transportation to doctor's visits, dietary supplements, and adjustments to account for lifestyle changes.

Developing a thorough financial plan that takes into account both direct and indirect expenses guarantees that people with Crohn's disease may concentrate on their health without having to worry about money. This plan needs to be reviewed and updated regularly because financial situations and healthcare demands might change over time.

CHAPITRE NINE

COPING WITH CROHN'S DISEASE: USEFUL ADVICE
Handling Crohn's Disease's Day-to-Day Difficulties

Managing the many obstacles that come with having Crohn's disease every day is necessary to keep things somewhat normal. Dietary management is one of the main issues. People who have Crohn's disease frequently have dietary sensitivity, necessitating a customized, limited diet. This calls for careful meal planning and knowledge of trigger foods that could make symptoms worse. Keeping a meal journal can be quite helpful in seeing trends and choosing the right nutrition.

Apart from food concerns, it's imperative to create a habit that places a high value on getting enough sleep. One typical symptom of Crohn's disease is fatigue, which can be made worse by sleep deprivation. A more regular sleep pattern, a comfortable sleeping environment, and the use of relaxation techniques can all improve general well-being. Since stress can lead to flare-ups, managing stress is just as crucial. Its effects can be lessened by implementing stress-reduction techniques including yoga, mindfulness, and meditation.

The secret to handling day-to-day difficulties is having effective communication with healthcare practitioners. Proactive healthcare is made possible by frequent check-ins and candid conversations regarding symptoms, prescriptions, and concerns. Creating a network of friends, family, and other Crohn's disease patients can also offer emotional support and a sense of belonging. Exchanging insights, advice, and coping techniques can empower others and build resilience in the face of day-to-day difficulties.

Crohn's Disease Travel: Charting Unknown Grounds

When traveling with Crohn's disease, it's important to prepare ahead and take precautions to make sure things go smoothly and reduce the chance of flare-ups. Finding and choosing travel locations with accessible medical facilities is one of the first tasks. Peace of mind can be attained by becoming familiar with the local medical system and having an emergency plan in place.

Careful packing is essential for people with Crohn's disease. It's crucial to always have a sufficient quantity of prescription drugs on hand. It is a good idea to bring along a travel-sized first aid kit that has basic supplies like painkillers, antidiarrheal pills, and any customized goods that a doctor may recommend. It's important to stay hydrated when traveling, and carrying a reusable water bottle will help guarantee that you have access to clean water.

When traveling, the timing and pace of activities are quite important. Making time for pauses and rest intervals facilitates moments of relaxation and lowers stress, which is frequently the cause of Crohn's disease symptoms. Traveling can be made more enjoyable by looking into modes of transportation that can meet certain needs, including toilets that are easily accessible.

Keeping a trip notebook can prove to be a beneficial instrument in monitoring symptoms and pinpointing possible triggers encountered while traveling. Thinking back on past trips can help with future travel arrangements and advance knowledge of managing Crohn's disease while traveling.

Work-Health Balancing: Techniques for Enhancing Professional Welfare

For those with Crohn's disease, juggling jobs and health is a delicate dance. It is essential to be transparent with employers on any potential adjustments and health needs. Creating a welcoming workplace that recognizes the erratic nature of Crohn's disease can enhance well-being in general.

Work schedule flexibility, remote work choices, and understanding coworkers can all reduce stress and make the working world more livable.

People with Crohn's disease must prioritize self-care during working hours. Short breaks for stretching, deep breathing exercises, or mindful activities might help promote a better work-life balance and higher productivity. It's also critical to design a workspace that meets workers' health needs, including convenient access to restrooms.

It's critical to include stress-reduction strategies throughout the workday. This could be quick breaks for quick meditation sessions, deep breathing techniques, or quick strolls. Burnout can be avoided and energy can be divided between job obligations and self-care by practicing proactive time management and goal-setting.

Creating a network of empathetic coworkers can help with emotional support and loneliness reduction. Providing coworkers with information on Crohn's disease, including its symptoms and potential obstacles, can promote empathy and establish a more welcoming work atmosphere. In the end, maintaining a commitment to prioritizing well-being in the workplace, self-advocacy, and constant communication are necessary to strike a balance between professional obligations and health demands.

CHAPTER TEN

TALES OF VICTORY: FIRSTHAND ACCOUNTS
Motivational Testimonials from People Overcoming Crohn's

Overcoming Crohn's disease is frequently an arduous path with many ups and downs. But woven throughout this battle is a tapestry of inspirational stories from people who have overcome the terrible enemy known as Crohn's disease. For individuals now negotiating the difficulties of the condition, these stories are rays of hope. One such person, Sarah, as we shall refer to her here, accepted the prognosis with steadfast resolve. Resilience characterized Sarah's path as she adopted a holistic approach to symptom management. Sarah was able to reduce her symptoms and regain her sense of power and purpose by combining medical treatments, dietary modifications, and a strong support network.

These stories highlight the resilience of the human spirit in the face of difficulty.

People with Crohn's disease share not only the medical struggles but also the mental and emotional strength needed to overcome it. These tales are linked to the significance of proactive self-care, in which people take responsibility for their health. These stories highlight the various approaches people have taken to overcome Crohn's disease, such as trying mindfulness exercises, investigating alternative therapies, or finding comfort in a caring community.

Readers are inspired by the wide range of strategies that have worked as they immerse themselves in these resilience stories. The experiences demonstrate that there is no one-size-fits-all approach, from adopting a customized pharmaceutical plan to trying out different meals. Instead, each person forges their special route to success. The stories promote a sense of reality and relatability by acknowledging the setbacks in addition to highlighting the successes. Through the combined voice of these stories, a potent testament to the resilience of the human spirit and its capacity to overcome the obstacles presented by Crohn's disease is shown.

Knowledge Acquired and Wisdom Exchanged:

In the context of conquering Crohn's disease, a multitude of insights and collective knowledge are revealed by the personal accounts of those who have encountered this strong foe. These observations not only provide direction for those who are coping with the illness at hand, but they also add to a body of knowledge that enhances medical professionals' comprehension of Crohn's disease.

Proactive communication with healthcare experts is a key lesson that is evident in all of these stories. People talk about the difficulties they've had figuring out possible side effects, dosage schedules, and treatment options. They discover the value of continuing honest and open communication with their healthcare staff via trial and error. The importance of people actively engaging in their healthcare journey by enquiring, seeking clarification, and speaking up for their well-being is emphasized by this shared wisdom.

The collective knowledge of those who have overcome Crohn's disease also heavily emphasizes dietary breakthroughs. People who experiment with different diets find that nutrition has a significant effect on managing their symptoms. Through the identification of trigger foods and the adoption of anti-inflammatory diets, these narratives highlight the relevance of nutrition as an adjunctive component within the treatment plan. People are encouraged by this collective wisdom to approach their food choices with inquiry and to be willing to modify them based on their unique experiences.

A recurrent issue is the significance of developing a strong support network. People all know the transformational power of seeking support from friends, family, and other Crohn's disease warriors in their hour of greatest need. This group's collective wisdom highlights the need to establish relationships within the community, whether via Internet forums or neighborhood support groups.

Through these shared stories, people find strength in their relationships with those who have experienced the subtleties of living with Crohn's disease, in addition to their resiliency.

In conclusion, these victories over Crohn's disease provide a wealth of knowledge on resilience, flexibility, and the significant benefits of a holistic approach to health. Every story adds to the growing body of knowledge on comprehending and treating this complicated illness, weaving together a tapestry of common experiences that can act as a lighthouse for those who are presently making their way.

CHAPTER ELEVEN

CONSIDERING THE FUTURE
Studies and Advancements in the Management of Crohn's Disease:

Promising prospects for the management of Crohn's disease exist due to continuous research and advances in treatment choices. To address the fundamental causes of Crohn's disease, researchers are investigating novel therapeutic methods as our understanding of the illness's underlying mechanisms advances. Treatments specific to each patient's genetic profile with Crohn's disease are becoming possible thanks to advances in precision medicine and genetic research.

The creation of biologics, or drugs made from living things, is one area of noteworthy advancement. By focusing on particular immune system pathways, these biologics help control the inflammatory response that is typical of Crohn's disease. Furthermore, research into microbiome-based treatments is accelerating as more people become aware of the complex connection between gut flora and Crohn's disease progression. The potential of probiotics, fecal microbiota transplantation, and other microbiome-targeted therapies to alleviate symptoms and restore a balanced gut microbiota is being studied.

Technological developments in medicine delivery are also improving therapeutic efficacy and reducing adverse effects. For example, nanotechnology is making it possible to deliver drugs to particular parts of the gastrointestinal tract with precision, improving treatment results. Additionally, the efficacy of novel drug classes and small molecules is being assessed in ongoing clinical trials, offering a range of alternatives to patients who have become intolerant to standard therapies.

The translation of scientific findings into practical treatment alternatives is accelerated by collaborations among researchers, pharmaceutical companies, and healthcare practitioners. Artificial intelligence and machine learning are being used to analyze large datasets, spot trends, and forecast treatment outcomes as technology develops. This data-driven strategy could completely change how Crohn's disease is managed by providing more individualized and accurate treatment plans.

In summary, a dynamic environment of research and innovation characterizes the treatment of Crohn's disease in the future. The combination of cutting-edge medication delivery technologies, microbiome science, and genetics is changing the therapeutic landscape and providing promise for more individualized and successful interventions for people with Crohn's disease.

Campaigning and Increasing Awareness:

To create a supportive atmosphere for those impacted by Crohn's disease, advocacy, and awareness-raising are crucial as we look to the future of the fight against this chronic condition. The goal of advocacy is to make people with Crohn's disease more vocal so that their demands are heard and laws are put in place to help them deal with the difficulties they encounter. These endeavors encompass both the social and political spheres, cultivating an awareness of the ramifications of Crohn's disease on persons and the criticality of easily accessible, reasonably priced healthcare.

The foundation of advocacy is increasing awareness, which involves debunking rumors and false information about Crohn's disease and spreading factual knowledge. Campaigns for public awareness, educational projects, and community engagement efforts help create a more knowledgeable public and lessen the stigma attached to chronic illnesses. These initiatives build a network of support for those living with Crohn's disease, allowing them to face their health journeys with dignity and resiliency. They do this by encouraging empathy and understanding.

Advocacy groups seek policies on the political front that improve access to high-quality healthcare, such as reasonably priced drugs and customized therapies for Crohn's disease. They work together with legislators, the pharmaceutical industry, and medical professionals to create laws that put the interests of people with Crohn's disease first. This lobbying is essential to guaranteeing that funds for study are allotted to progress remedies and enhance the general well-being of those impacted.

Social media and internet platforms offer strong instruments for advocacy and awareness efforts in the digital age. People can interact with a worldwide community committed to advocating for Crohn's disease, exchange personal stories, and establish connections with others going through comparable difficulties. These forums act as sparks for public opinion, research funding, and support mobilization.

In the future, persistent advocacy and awareness campaigns will be crucial to creating a society that is kind and knowledgeable and that gives people with Crohn's disease a sense of empowerment. The future appears to hold the possibility of a more inclusive and supportive environment for individuals navigating the difficulties of Crohn's disease through the promotion of understanding, the advocacy of policy reforms, and the utilization of digital platforms.

Promoting Hope and Adaptability:

For those facing the difficulties of a chronic illness, cultivating optimism and perseverance is crucial in the fight against Crohn's disease. Having a chronic condition can be physically and emotionally exhausting, therefore it's important to keep a positive mindset for general well-being. The treatment of Crohn's disease in the future must place a high priority on holistic strategies that promote the mental and emotional well-being of those who have the illness in addition to treating their physical symptoms.

The development of resilience is greatly aided by psychosocial interventions such as counseling, support groups, and mental health resources. Healthcare professionals are incorporating mental health assistance into the entire treatment plan for patients with Crohn's disease, acknowledging the psychosocial effects of chronic illness. This method stresses the value of a comprehensive care plan while acknowledging the connections between mental and physical health.

Education initiatives that emphasize stress management, mindfulness, and coping techniques are increasingly important to the therapy of Crohn's disease. Through the development of resilience skills, these programs enable individuals to approach the uncertainty of their health journey with optimism. Furthermore, mentoring programs and peer support networks link people going through comparable struggles, creating a sense of belonging and mutual understanding.

Hope and resilience are being fostered by technological breakthroughs as well. Without regard to location, telehealth services, online support communities, and health applications offer easily accessible means for people to interact with medical experts and other patients. These online forums provide areas for exchanging coping mechanisms, success stories, and motivational tales in addition to providing helpful assistance.

Future Crohn's disease management strategies will place a higher priority on people's emotional health because they understand that resilience is a crucial tool for overcoming the challenges of managing a chronic illness. In a future where people with Crohn's disease not only manage their symptoms but also thrive with resilience and hope, the healthcare sector may contribute by integrating psychosocial support, educational resources, and technology-driven solutions.